ARTEM KUDELIA PHD

Beyond Psychiatry

Exploring Anti-Psychiatry Method

This book is not intended to substitute for professional medical or psychological advice or treatment if necessary. It is recommended that you consult the appropriate specialist if you require medical, psychological, or any other professional assistance or treatment.

If you are experiencing severe symptoms of a serious mental or physical health condition, the advice provided in this book may not be suitable or sufficient for you. If you have not already done so, it is strongly advised that you seek the guidance and collaboration of an experienced mental health professional or medical practitioner.

If your symptoms or issues worsen while reading this book, it is important to stop reading immediately and seek help from a qualified healthcare professional.

The author, publishers, and any subsequent distributors of this work are not responsible for any errors, assumptions, or interpretations made while utilizing this information. Readers have the sole responsibility of understanding and making use of this information.

First edition

This book was professionally typeset on Reedsy.
Find out more at reedsy.com

Contents

Acknowledgments

I would like to express my gratitude to my psychology and psychotherapy teachers, who have opened the path and laid a solid foundation of knowledge. Furthermore, I extend my immense appreciation to patients, colleagues, friends, and all individuals who directly or indirectly contributed to the writing of this book.

BONUS: Get Your Free Resources Now

I'm excited to share a **free eBook** and **exclusive access** to **psychological resources** with you. To get started, scan the QR code or visit psychemaster.com/beyond-psychiatry

What You'll Get:

- **Free eBook**: Explore advanced psychotherapeutic techniques and approaches that complement the insights.
- **Interactive Learning**: Engage with exercises and quizzes to solidify your understanding of complex theories.
- **Latest Research**: Stay updated with the most recent findings in the field of psychotherapy and integrative therapy approaches.
- **Continuous Support**: Get consistent tips, strategies, and motivation to assist you in staying focused and excelling in your studies and practice.

Maximize your understanding of psychotherapy!

Antipsychiatry

Antipsychiatry is not a comprehensive practical methodology for therapeutic work but rather a philosophy. It offers a fresh perspective on the world of mental deviations, presenting new "windows" through which we can gain a deeper understanding of the reality of psychological disorders.

To some professionals, the ideas of antipsychiatry and its proponents may seem insane and disconnected from reality. However, it is important to remember that the concept of illness is always based on a general understanding of health and normalcy. Yet, one must not forget that the notion of normalcy is not static. It changes in accordance with the spirit of the times. What is considered normal in one culture may be perceived as madness in another.

Recognizing the relativity of our notions of normalcy, it is crucial to acknowledge that those individuals who, from our perspective, may appear insane are not always so in the grand scheme of things. Countless examples can be cited by recalling the biographies of various renowned scientists who exhibited peculiarities in their behavior, speech, and thinking.

The ideas of antipsychiatry began to flourish in the mid-20th century, largely due to the efforts of Ronald Laing. Some of his colleagues embraced this new wave in psychiatry and creatively developed its principles.

Ronald David Laing

Ronald David Laing (1927–1989) was born in Glasgow, Scotland, in the United Kingdom. He was the only child of David Park MacNair Laing and Amelia Glen Laing. Laing believed that his childhood was unhappy due to his emotionally restrained and non-affectionate mother. He received his primary education at Hutchesons' Boys' Grammar School in Glasgow. Laing developed a strong interest in philosophy at a young age and read the works of famous philosophers such as Plato, Aristotle, Sophocles, Aeschylus, and others. He was also musically talented and engaged in singing and music, becoming a licentiate of the Royal Academy of Music and a member of the Royal Music Society in 1944–1945.

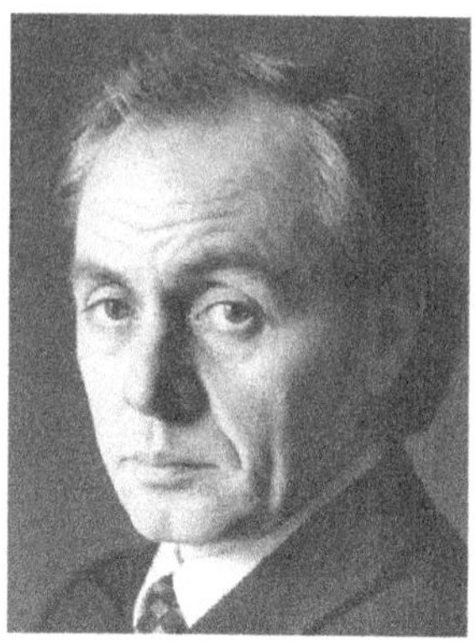

Ronald Laing

From 1945 to 1951, Laing studied medicine at the University of Glasgow while also working as a hospital orderly in a psychiatric ward. This experience greatly influenced his choice of future specialization, which would be neurology. During his studies, Laing's attention was drawn to ethical questions regarding the relationship between philosophy and medicine. He also became part of a group of amateur researchers who practiced hypnotic suggestion for experimental purposes.

Laing had a passionate interest in sports as well. He engaged in tennis, mountaineering, croquet, and track and field athletics.

He underwent an internship in the neurosurgical department of the Gartnavel Royal Hospital under the guidance of former field surgeon Joe Schorstein, who introduced him to the works of philosophers and psychotherapists such as Kant, Husserl, Kierkegaard, Sartre, Wittgenstein, Freud, Jung, and others.

From 1951 to 1953, Laing served as a military psychiatrist in the Royal Army Medical Corps. In his work as a psychiatrist, he strove to establish a confidential rapport with his patients.

Through this trusting relationship, he was able to help many patients regain their connection with life. Rumors circulated that during his service, Laing preferred the company of his patients over that of his colleagues. It was during this time that he gradually developed the belief that madness was more of a philosophical question than a medical symptom. According to Laing, understanding the world of the mentally ill, accepting them "as they are," and engaging in peaceful interactions could initiate unique psychotherapeutic processes within the patient's psyche. From Laing's perspective, madness could be seen not merely as a symptom but as a personal characteristic.

During his military service, Laing met Anne Hann, with whom he began a relationship. The young couple soon got married, and they went on to have five children.

After leaving the army, Laing started working as a psychiatrist at the Gartnavel Royal Psychiatric Hospital in Glasgow, where he conducted one of his experiments with mentally ill patients. This experiment, known as the "noisy room," took place from 1954 to 1955. In this experiment, both the staff and the patients at the clinic remained in their usual attire and engaged in regular interactions and daily activities. Laing aimed to simulate a normal psychological environment, which he believed was a crucial therapeutic factor in working with patients. The experiment proved successful, and indeed, Laing's approach yielded constructive results.

In 1956, Ronald Laing, along with his family, moved to London where he took up a position as a senior registrar at the Tavistock Clinic. He also underwent comprehensive psychoanalytic training at the Institute of Psychoanalysis under the guidance of Donald Woods Winnicott.

In 1958, together with Aaron Esterson, Laing embarked on

an in-depth study of families with schizophrenic patients, aiming to uncover the underlying causes of the illness. He began to view schizophrenia not as an individual's disease but as a "knot" within the family system. Laing's term "knot" can be understood as a specific interconnection between the individual and the social group to which they belong. In this sense, schizophrenia started to be interpreted as a problem of integrating the individual into the social environment. The research conducted by Laing and Esterson enabled them to identify typical profiles of the schizophrenic patients' father and mother. In such families, the father is often weak and submissive, while the mother is cold and domineering.

In 1960, Laing opened his private psychoanalytic practice. That same year, one of his most famous books, "The Divided Self," was published, receiving numerous positive reviews and accolades in medical journals. Although the book initially did not gain immediate recognition, it eventually became a full-fledged bestseller. Laing begins his book with the definitions of the "existential-phenomenological foundation of science and personality" and "existential-phenomenological understanding of psychosis." He introduces the term "ontological insecurity," which forms the basis for his model of schizophrenia, as an attempt to preserve the unstable "self" through internal fragmentation and the creation of an external false mask.

In 1961, his second book, "Self and Others," was published, serving as a conceptual and ideological continuation of his previous work.

In 1962, Laing assumed leadership of the Langham Clinic in London.

Laing became one of the psychiatrists who worked and wrote in the spirit of anti-psychiatry philosophy. The central thesis of this philosophy suggests that mental illness is a myth created by society to control individuals who deviate from the majority.

Starting in the mid-1960s, Laing began to appear frequently on television where he presented his views. He hosted a television program dedicated to topics such as madness, health, and family. Laing's rebellious philosophy eventually made him an idol among British youth.

While Laing embraced existentialism and anti-psychiatry in his ideological and philosophical realms, which largely informed his literary works, in practice, in his work with patients, he employed various methods of psychotherapy such as behavioral therapy, gestalt therapy, and existential therapy. As a result, his approach can be considered eclectic.

In 1964, while in the USA, Laing met Timothy Leary, a prominent advocate for the use of LSD. Intrigued by Leary's ideas, he returned to the United Kingdom and began applying LSD to his patients. It is worth noting that, at that time, LSD was not yet prohibited and was seen as one of the therapeutic tools.

In 1965, together with Esterson, Laing established an experimental community for schizophrenic individuals called "Kingsley Hall." The clinic's work was based on Laing's experimental experience with the "noisy room" in Cooper's Community, "Villa 21," and a kibbutz for schizophrenics in Israel that Esterson had studied. At Kingsley Hall, there was no hierarchy, and there was no formal division between doctors and patients. This community existed for five years before it was closed. In many ways, Laing's experiment holds a significant place in the history of psychiatry and has yielded some constructive results. However, due to its extravagance, it did not find widespread acceptance in the field of psychiatry.

The personality of the schizophrenic was neither suppressed

nor confined. To some extent, Laing perceived schizophrenia as a psychedelic journey induced by the ingestion of hallucinogens, which could end well in the presence of comfortable and balanced conditions and warm emotional support from the environment. In this regard, Laing partially adopted the practices of psychedelic psychotherapists of that time who believed that the administration of psychedelic substances during psychotherapy could bring about substantial constructive changes in patients, provided there was a good rapport and a supportive relationship between the therapist and the patient.

In the second half of the 1960s, Laing separated from his first wife and married a German woman named Jutta Wernicke, with whom he had three more children—two boys and one girl.

In the early 1970s, the book "Laing and Antipsychiatry," edited by R. Boyers, was published, solidifying the "brand" of antipsychiatry not only with David Cooper, who published the work "Psychiatry and Antipsychiatry" in 1967, but also with Laing.

In 1971, Laing embarked on a journey to Ceylon (now Sri Lanka) with his wife and two children, where he spent two months studying Buddhism, which was gaining popularity worldwide. He then traveled to India, where he explored various Hindu practices, received initiation into the cult of the goddess Kali, and studied Sanskrit. He attended lectures by Buddhist Lama Govinda, who was Timothy Leary's guru.

A year later, Laing returned to London and went on a lecture tour of the United States in 1972. During his time in the US, Laing met Elizabeth Fehr, who applied the technique of "rebirthing psychodrama" in her practice. The goal of this technique was to re-experience the birth process and release symptoms through the expression of repressed emotions.

Laing became interested in this practice, adopted it, and began using it with his patients from 1973 on. This technique shares similarities with Stanislav Grof's holotropic breathwork, which was also actively developing at that time, especially after the prohibition on the use of LSD in clinical settings.

In the 1970s, Ronald Laing published works such as "Knots" (1971), "Do You Love Me?" (1976), "Facts of Life" (1976), and "Conversations with Children" (1978). In 1985, he published his autobiography titled "Wisdom, Madness, and Folly."

In the 1980s, Laing separated from his second wife and met another German woman, Sue Zanghell, with whom he had another son. However, his relationship with Zanghell lasted only one and a half years.

Towards the end of his life, Laing entered into a relationship with his secretary, Margaret, who gave birth to his son in 1988.

Laing passed away from a heart attack that occurred while playing tennis at the French resort town of Saint-Tropez.

Laing wrote about psychological states such as ontological certainty and uncertainty about the self. Ontological certainty about the self can create a foundation for deriving pleasure from interpersonal connections. On the other hand, ontological uncertainty only breeds preoccupation with one's own safety, imposes limitations on social interactions, and hinders genuine satisfaction.

Laing wrote about three forms of anxiety stemming from ontological uncertainty about the self. These are:

1. **Engulfment**: This form of anxiety is associated with fear of any kind of relationship, both external with others and internal with oneself. The individual is frightened by contact, the expression of warm emotions, attachment,

and so on. (This anxiety can be referred to as a schizoid conditionally.)

2. **Fissure**: In this form, individuals experience and undergo an existential vacuum, a sense of inner emptiness. Complete contact with external reality is perceived as a potentially traumatizing process capable of generating only problems. Reality, other people, and social events are seen as persecuting the individual. (This anxiety can be conditionally termed paranoid.)

3. **Petrification**: According to Laing, petrification can manifest in three forms:

- A feeling of terror that causes a person to "freeze." It is a particular psychological pain that, once experienced, renders the person insensitive to emotional relationships.
- Fear of being transformed from a living person into an automaton, a robot, or a stone. It is anxiety regarding being used, transformed into a routine element of the world, and preoccupied with external formalities.
- Fear of turning others into "stones," perceiving others as objects, and disregarding their feelings. (This anxiety can be conditionally termed psychopathic.)

Laing discussed two types of personalities in relation to their connection with the bodily aspect. These types do not represent the polarity of mental health and illness; each has its own advantages and disadvantages. They are:

1. **Embodied personality**: By an embodied personality, he

meant an individual who has a connection with their body, sensations, and feelings and considers themselves alive. They sense that they consist of flesh, blood, and bones. For such individuals, mind and body are inseparable. However, the split within them can occur in other situations. In certain situations, an embodied personality may be much more vulnerable than an unembodied one. Embodiment of personality does not guarantee protection against anxiety, stress, and other mental disorders. (This type is most closely related to the concept of epileptoid personality.)

2. **Unembodied personality**: Such a personality perceives itself separately from its body, which is seen as one of the objects in the external world. The individual becomes an external observer, a dissociated critic, detached from emotions and experiences. (This type of personality is most closely related to the concept of schizoid personality.)

Laing presents his view of personality as a specific norm and the culmination of various psychic mechanisms at work, such as repression, displacement, projection, introjection, splitting, and so on. Some functions of these defense mechanisms can be considered constructive, leading to a balanced control of the individual, while other functions can create destructive experiences that significantly alienate the individual from the structure of existence. Laing believed that the prevailing notion in psychiatry that patients should be changed into inanimate objects rather than accepted as living human beings perpetuates the illness that is diligently being treated. According to him, psychotherapy should strive to restore the fullness of warmth in communication between individuals through their interconnectedness.

One of the terms frequently used by Laing was "metanoia." In Ancient Greek, it translates as a change of mind, a reevaluation, or a change of thought. It signifies a shift in perception accompanied by regret and repentance. In religion, "metanoia" signifies "repentance." In analytical psychology, Carl Jung borrowed this term from Heraclitus and used it as a synonym for another term, "enantiodromia," referring to the process of something transitioning into its diametrical opposite. Laing himself defined metanoia as a schizophrenic psychosis that involves a process of testing and potential rebirth, capable of leading to the true essence of one's personality. Other psychiatrists associated with the anti-psychiatry movement, particularly David Cooper, held similar views.

In his theories, Laing sometimes leaned toward an ultra-radical anti-psychiatric position, explaining that in the context of human socialization, one's consciousness becomes mystified, causing individuals to enter a world of social hallucinations that most people call reality. What is commonly referred to as health is, in fact, a variety of madness that is not easily cured. In this conviction of Laing's, we can see the influence of Buddhism with its philosophy of the illusory nature of the world, the need for enlightenment, and transcending the cycle of samsara. Another strong anti-psychiatric belief of Laing's was that psychiatrists could learn more about the inner world and specific experiences from schizophrenics than the other way around. This belief was also shared by another advocate of the American anti-psychiatry movement, Frank Farrelly, the creator of provocative therapy, who commented during his seminars that his best teachers were his patients.

American psychologist Kirk Schneider claimed that Laing

described psychosis as if he were "leading a team of researchers who had visited an abandoned island of psychotics." Kirk believed that Laing was a pioneer in his field. To some extent, he can be compared to the French physician Pinel, the founder of psychiatry in France, who became widely known for his reforms in the treatment of the mentally ill in clinics. Thanks to Pinel, patients with mental disorders were unchained, and he also implemented hospital regulations and doctor visits. Schneider also referred to Laing as an astronaut of consciousness.

Laing wrote in "The Phenomenology of Experience": "If the human race survives, future men will, I suspect, look back on our enlightened epoch as the time when a great many certainties were known to be uncertain and the multitude of dogmas that had been regarded as axiomatic for thousands of years were gradually and sometimes painfully withdrawn. We, of course, cannot feel this future in our bones, but it can be anticipated intellectually."

David Graham Cooper

David Cooper (1931–1986) was one of the creators of the anti-psychiatry movement in psychiatry. He was born in Cape Town and received his medical education there. In 1955, he moved to Paris, where he found his wife, and soon after to London, where he opened a private practice and worked in several medical institutions. One of the significant encounters in Cooper's life occurred in 1958 when he met Ronald Laing, who shared most of his professional views. They began a fruitful collaboration, and in 1964, they co-authored the book "Reason and Violence: A Decade of Sartre's Creative Work."

In 1965, Cooper participated in the establishment of the therapeutic community "Kingsley Hall" founded by Laing. In 1967, Cooper published the book "Psychiatry and Anti-Psychiatry," which formally became the first comprehensive work to introduce the term "anti-psychiatry" and discuss various philosophical concepts related to this movement in psychiatry. Cooper also wrote works such as "The Death of the Family," "The Grammar of Living," and "The Language of Madness."

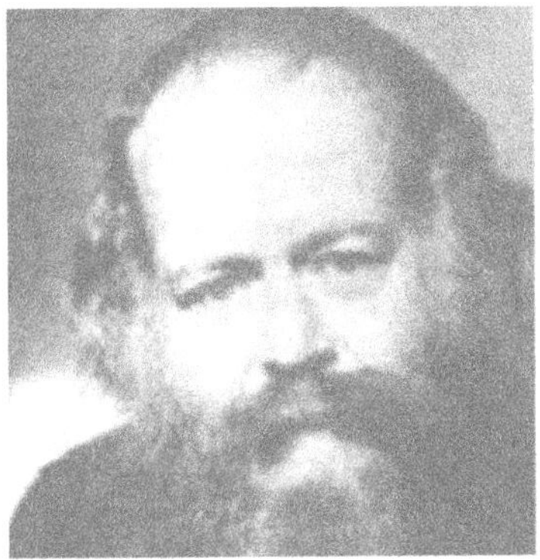

David Cooper

Cooper advocated for a social model of the development of psychotic disorders, believing that symptoms arise in individuals through socialization. It is primarily Cooper who can be considered the person who popularized the term "anti-psychiatry" in scientific discourse, largely due to his rejection of the clinical psychiatric treatment methods that existed at the time. In addition to the philosophical concept of anti-psychiatry, Cooper was influenced by Marxism, existentialism, and French structuralism and post-structuralism. Cooper held radical and aggressive anti-psychiatric convictions that not only called for reforms in medicine but also provoked revolutionary sentiments. He believed that we were living in a pre-revolutionary period and that the revolution itself should start with a "revolution of madness," that is, the dismantling of psychiatric institutions as they existed before.

In addition to the "revolution of madness," Cooper advocated for a "revolution of love," the liberation of society from puritanical sexual morality, considering the "bed" as one of the secret weapons of the revolution. He saw the potential in a comprehensive social revolution, reformation, and dismantling of the foundations of bourgeois society. The "revolution of madness" was seen by him as the initial link that could trigger further processes of total social transformation.

Cooper developed the concept of "the grammar of the political," which is a specific grammar of power and influence within the context of the psychic and social space. This concept is divided into four levels.

1. **The micro-political level of the inner space of the individual:** Psychic and physical experiences can be seen as political acts. In other words, any form of psychological or physical disorder is a metaphorical expression of a structural problem of communication existing within the group to which the individual belongs. The interconnection between external social aspects and profound internal aspects is explored. To some extent, Cooper attempts to consider the world of an individual's inner experiences as a smaller fractal in relation to larger social processes, highlighting the interdependence of different internal processes and their structural orderliness. This is the internal psychic level.

2. **The micro-political level of the family:** The family system, in which the individual matures, shapes a specific structure of experience that potentially becomes a cause for internal conflicts within a person who does not feel the need for close fusion with others. This level pertains to family systems.

3. **The micro-political level of confrontational groups:** This level encompasses various social institutions and organizations that replicate the functioning structure of the family. A child goes to school, attends college, visits hospitals, and serves in the army—all these social organizations are closely interconnected on a structural level with how the family system functions and what profound values it propagates. This level relates to larger organizational systems.

4. **Macro-political level:** Determines the functioning of all social organizations in society to some extent. The transformation at the macro-political level can bring about changes at all other levels of social and psychological existence.

We will provide commentary and note that, in general, the conditioning of the levels occurs from bottom to top, meaning from the fourth level to the first. However, despite this, all levels are closely interrelated, so not only does the greater condition the smaller, but the smaller also influences the greater, being an integral part of it. It is important to reiterate that this model is best understood through the lens of Mandelbrot's fractal concept, which suggests that a smaller fragment of a system symbolically reflects the structure of a larger fragment and exists in a specific form of interdependence with it. Thus, Cooper presents a model that considers the sphere of the political and the psychic within a particular holistic continuum, which is a relatively rare phenomenon in psychological and psychiatric models. Typically, these spheres are not integrated into comprehensive concepts and models in most personality theories.

Cooper believed that the structure of the family and domestic life conditioned individuals to always be part of a social group and discouraged solitude. Any manifestation of personal autonomy can be a blow to the organization of the family system. Cooper was convinced that madness is a movement away from a familial mode of existence.

Contact and connection with other individuals are encouraged, as is the pursuit of autonomous existence, where the individual can function as a self-sufficient personality. At the very least, he pointed out certain values actively declared in society that proclaim the integrity of the family system as a criterion of normalcy and adequacy for an individual.

He also believed that schizophrenic disorders were a consequence of the suppression of personality in society. This suppression occurs through the imposition of stereotypical values. Unwillingness to conform to the majority's values is perceived as madness and is not only criticized on a moral level but also subjected to social and institutional pressure. Contemporary psychiatry is a clear example of this.

Cooper, to a large extent, equated madness with rebellion and dissidence. In this sense, a madman acts as a kind of revolutionary whose activity is directed not outwardly toward the social world but toward psychic experiences. In this, we must note Cooper's originality of thought, as he truly directed attention to mental disorders, drawing analogies between internal psychic processes and external politics.

Both Cooper and Laing believed that schizophrenia in an individual was a vivid manifestation of a crisis within the social group they belonged to. The need to break free from the shackles of social pressure finds expression in various psychotic symptoms.

Cooper expressed rather radical convictions that if the structure of family functioning, as accepted in our society, could be destroyed, we would liberate individuals from a behavioral model that potentially triggers schizophrenic symptoms.

He also believed that the schizophrenic process could be a peculiar attempt to regain lost wholeness.

Like Laing, Cooper used the term "metanoia" and perceived it as a form of movement between four states: eknoia, paranoia, noia, and antinoia. In Cooper's understanding, they are interpreted as follows:

1. **Eknoia:** This is the condition of the majority of people who live in society and conform to its rules and norms. Living in a state of eknoia is a constant way of annihilating one's true self, rejecting it for the sake of certain social ideals that are imprinted on a person from early childhood without choice. Sooner or later, the state of eknoia can provoke a deep rebellion within a person, a realization that something is fundamentally wrong or incorrect. However, being devoid of the cards on how to leave one's established place, individuals mostly begin to exhibit certain anxieties and eventually psychotic symptoms.

2. **Paranoia:** In a state of paranoia, individuals become uncertain about the correctness of social organization. They begin to realize that their profound essence is suppressed, and they are unable to fully be who they truly are.

3. **Noia:** In this state, individuals may experience intense

depression and sadness due to the process of separating themselves from their social group. The old mask has not yet been fully removed, and the new one has not yet formed, but the irreversibility of specific personal transformations is already felt.

4. **Antinoia:** This state is the transcendence of one's self, the destruction of one's former self, and its complete transmutation and transformation. It is a state that brings the individual closer to a transcendent experience. The psychospiritual journey may be perceived as a form of madness, but in this case, we witness the relativity of such madness. A person who has entered this state may perceive individuals in the state of eknoia as mad.

Each of these states is experienced by an individual sequentially. Each element of the model represents a progression culminating in the fourth stage. With each stage, there is a gradual reshaping and restructuring of the personality.

To a large extent, the process of transitioning from eknoia to antinoia can be perceived as a continuum of a child's impressions during the process of birth. Eknoia is perceived as a state of fusion with the womb, paranoia as the period of the onset of labor contractions along the birth canal, noia as the process of exiting the womb, detachment, and cutting of the umbilical cord, and antinoia as the existence of the individual outside the womb. If we consider Cooper's model in this way, we can note its strong resemblance to Stanislav Grof's model of basic perinatal matrices (BPM). In any case, we must acknowledge that both authors delve into certain profound impressions in the human unconscious using different maps of description.

David Cooper, following the example of Tommaso Campanella and his utopia "The City of the Sun," constructed his ideas about the ideals of a therapeutic society in which the model of solitary existence and the model of interconnectedness with other members of society could coexist harmoniously. Cooper believed that only when an individual learns to be autonomous and experience solitude can they fully engage with others.

Despite the somewhat utopian nature of these models, Cooper managed to conduct an experiment in which he observed the functioning of his "therapeutic society." This project was called "Villa 21" and operated for four years in one of the wards at Shenley Hospital.

The project involved patients between the ages of 15 and 30 with symptoms of schizophrenia, psychopathy, and other personality disorders. The aim of the experiment was to attempt to prove that the classical system of functioning in psychiatric institutions, characterized by rigid regulations and repressive modes of intervention, is not necessary and, moreover, can contribute to the deterioration of patients' conditions. During the experiment, patients were not confined within the usual boundaries traditionally seen in psychiatric institutions and actively participated in assisting and supporting one another. The democratic system of functioning within the ward and the equal relationships between patients and therapists did not compromise the quality of the ward's work. Positive results were obtained, indicating that the adopted structure of relationships is not a significant and obligatory attribute of the ward's functioning. The experience gained from "Villa 21" served as the foundation for the future collaborative experiment of Laing and Cooper in their therapeutic community, "Kingsley Hall."

Unfortunately, the progressive beliefs and long-term experiments of Laing and Cooper did not find widespread application. It can be assumed that their philosophical and practical findings await their time and will unfold to their full potential.

Thomas Szasz

Thomas Szasz (1920–2012) was a renowned American psychiatrist, professor of psychiatry, and a prominent figure in the anti-psychiatry movement. He was born in Budapest and was the younger of two sons in a Jewish family. His father was involved in private entrepreneurship. While attending school, Szasz demonstrated diligence as a student and excelled in sports. In 1938, the Szasz family moved to Cincinnati, USA, where Thomas enrolled in college at the university, specializing in the study of physics. In 1941, he completed his bachelor's degree in physics and decided to pursue a new specialization in medicine at the same university. He completed his education in 1944 and entered an internship program. In 1945, he received his medical degree. He then studied psychoanalytic therapy at the Chicago Institute of Psychoanalysis.

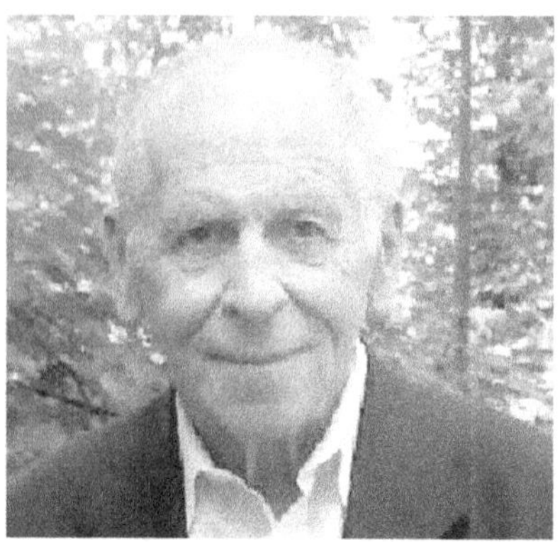

Thomas Szasz

Szasz's primary teacher in psychoanalysis was Franz Alexander, the founder of psychosomatic psychoanalysis, whose views significantly influenced Szasz's immersion in the scientific aspects of psychotherapy. Szasz's early scientific articles focused on psychosomatics, specifically symptoms such as hypersalivation, alopecia, constipation, and diarrhea. In 1951, Szasz obtained specialization in psychiatry and also got married. In 1954, he was drafted into military service during the Korean War. In 1956, he became a professor of psychiatry at Syracuse University, a position he held for the rest of his life. Prior to 1956, Szasz's work primarily dealt with issues of psychosomatics and classical psychoanalysis. In 1957, his first book, "Pain and Pleasure: A Study of Bodily Sensations," was published. In 1966, "The Myth of Mental Illness" was published, followed by "The Manufacture of Madness" in 1970. In these latter two books, which made Szasz particularly popular, he actively developed the philosophy of anti-psychiatry, providing a multifaceted historical analysis of it. In 1971, the American Humanist Academy awarded him the title of "Humanist of the Year."

Alongside Laing and Cooper, Szasz is one of the key activists in the anti-psychiatry movement. In his work, he paid significant attention to criticizing the functional structure of psychiatric care, arguing that political systems encourage the use of psychiatry as a punitive social instrument. He fought for the mental rights of individuals, believing that everyone has the right to govern their own mind and body as they see fit, both in terms of internal mental processes and external political matters. Szasz was a liberal and democrat who advocated for the fight for one's rights and ridiculed the absurdity of various social institutions' organizations.

In his book "The Myth of Mental Illness," Szasz comments that we cannot speak of a mental disorder as something real since we cannot directly observe what exactly happens within a person's psyche. In this view, Szasz aligns to a large extent with the philosophy of behaviorism proposed by B.F. Skinner and the concept of the "black box," which refers to certain internal processes that, for the most part, cannot be objectively investigated. Behaviorists aimed to exclude all unobservable mental processes from the realm of research. Unfortunately, this position ultimately led to the almost complete disappearance of behaviorism in its pure form. It is worth noting that Szasz wrote his main works at a time when neurophysiological diagnostics had not yet reached sufficient development. At that time, the scientist could afford not to rely on objective data, such as magnetic resonance imaging, which is capable of qualitatively describing the neurophysiological aspects of mental states and experiences. Szasz's disregard for numerous scientific data obtained through objective research on various disorders discredits his philosophical position. Unfortunately, until the end of his life, Szasz defended ideas that were formed in the late 1950s and early 1960s.

Like Laing and Cooper, Szasz expressed radical anti-psychiatric beliefs and argued that the concept of mental illness should be entirely removed from the classification of clinical medicine. Szasz then shifted to his understanding of the psychiatric institution, stating that it primarily exists as a political instrument and perpetuates the myth of mental illness to maintain positions of power and influence. Szasz even believed that psychiatry had become a parody of medicine and had become something akin to a separate state religion that dictates and predetermines the criteria of normality and abnormality at its own discretion. Michel Foucault, in his 1961 book "Madness and Civilization: A History of Insanity in the Age of Reason," shared Szasz's opinion regarding the dubious authenticity of psychiatry as a genuine science. An interesting observation made by the professor was regarding drug addiction, stating that drug addicts are persecuted in a similar manner to how Jews, Gypsies, witches, representatives of sexual minorities, and others were persecuted in different countries in the past.

Szasz expressed support for the following ideas:

- **Presumption of sanity:** Sanity and insanity should be determined through legal methods, with the right to appeal. A person is presumed sane until proven otherwise.

- **Right to suicide:** Szasz believes that suicide is an expression of personal choice, and the state should not impede it.

- **Abolition of the insanity defense:** According to Szasz, the determination of sanity or insanity by psychiatrists in court should be discontinued. He believes that such assessments are irrelevant to objective reality. By fulfilling this social function, the psychiatrist resembles a priest who condemns and judges.

- **Abolition of involuntary hospitalization:** Involuntary hospitalization, in Szasz's view, is a gross violation of individual rights. In the documentary film "Psychiatry: An Industry of Death," released in 2006, Szasz expressed his opinion that any form of involuntary hospitalization is a crime against humanity.

- **Personal right to drug use:** Szasz considered drug use to be a victimless crime. He also believed that addiction is not a disease. The medical concepts of addiction have no objective relation to reality. The use of substances that alter consciousness is an expression of individual freedom of choice. Substance dependence itself can be seen as a specific social ritual. Examples of this can be found in cultures where the use of consciousness-altering substances is a distinct cultural characteristic that has been present in society for many centuries and even millennia.

Szasz directed his rebellion and protest against the state institution of psychiatry, commenting that his philosophy often has no relation to the psychiatrists, psychotherapists, psychologists, and social workers who practice privately.

Behind Szasz's excessive, sometimes ultraradical, and scientifically unfounded approach to treating the mentally ill, we can trace his deep intention to defend personal freedom, fight for equality, and protect true moral values.

Pathopsychological Profiles and Anti-psychiatric Forms of Psychotherapy

It is important to emphasize from the outset that anti-psychiatric therapy is not merely a set of specific methods but rather a philosophy embraced by the psychotherapist in their practice. It is quite challenging to speak about the specific effectiveness of this therapeutic approach for patients, especially those who do not suffer from severe mental illnesses. It should be understood that in this case, the therapist's personality and the various instrumental practices they intend to employ in their work will play a significant role. However, one can observe a general pattern in the application of anti-psychiatric philosophy towards patients with different pathopsychological profiles.

Hysteroid Profile

Individuals with a hysteroid profile tend to adore indulging in the therapist's philosophical inclinations in order to receive positive feedback and, in turn, become the center of attention. Naturally, if the therapist's philosophical "credo" possesses a certain eccentricity that sets their therapeutic approach apart from others, hysteroids can readily embrace this game and become deeply involved in it. It is important to note that hysteroid personalities are often indifferent to the specific means by which attention is attracted. The therapist's profound conviction in the validity of an eccentric philosophy and therapy can be perceived by the patient as a peculiar and specific form of indulging their neurotic behavior. Therefore, the anti-psychiatric style of working with patients with a hysteroid personality profile should be applied in a measured and moderate manner. Only the proper combination of theory and practice in this case can bring about constructive changes in the patient.

Paranoid Profile

In my opinion, it is better not to apply the anti-psychiatric approach when working with paranoid patients. Most likely, a paranoid patient will construct their own specific and exaggerated paranoid reality based on the therapist's philosophy and behavior, which is unlikely to benefit them. Paranoids see deception everywhere. The likelihood of perceiving this "deception" in the therapist's behavior, who practices the philosophy of anti-psychiatry, will significantly increase in their eyes. Paranoid patients are not particularly fond of eccentric therapists or eccentric psychotherapeutic methods. This must be kept in mind.

Psychopathic Profile

A psychopathic patient may be inclined to play games of anti-psychiatry with the therapist. However, it should not be forgotten that any game involving a psychopathic individual is a game of predator and prey. When engaging in the game, the psychopath will clearly aim to outsmart the therapist. There is no need to indulge in the illusion that the profound philosophical meaning of anti-psychiatric therapy can emotionally touch a psychopath. They simply do not require it. Therefore, in the context of this profile, it is also necessary to state the complete inapplicability of this therapeutic philosophy.

Obsessive-Compulsive Profile

For patients with an obsessive-compulsive profile, the variety of anti-psychiatric philosophy can play a positive role when the instrumental aspects of therapeutic work are applied correctly. The excessive pedantry of such patients, combined with the therapist's appropriate methods, can provide the patient with confidence in their abilities. They may perceive the obsessions inherent in their personality as unique character traits that have not fully found proper social embodiment. In this case, practices aimed at redefining the meaning of the patient's actions can be particularly effective. A significant change in their attitude towards certain neurotic behaviors can serve as powerful support for the patient to develop self-confidence and create a more constructive self-image. Naturally, this will activate positive therapeutic psychodynamics within the individual. Therefore, for this particular personality profile, we recommend the application of anti-psychiatric theory and practice as needed, according to the patient's personality and the appropriateness of the therapeutic context.

Schizoid Profile

Depending on various psychodynamic factors, schizoid individuals will react differently to the practice of anti-psychiatric philosophy. A schizoid person experiences a need for detachment and dissociation from various conventional social routines and is often capable of creating interest-based clubs for fellow schizoids. Anti-psychiatric philosophy accommodates the idiosyncrasies of the patient, allowing them to perceive their symptoms not as deviations from the norm but as alternative versions of normality that can be accepted as given. Therefore, if this type of practical philosophy is applied to a schizoid individual, certain aspects of their personality will undergo constructive changes. If the right notes can be found within the schizoid's soul, working with anti-psychiatric philosophy and practice can create a powerful rapport that potentially becomes a precursor to constructive changes in the patient's personality.

Epileptoid Profile

Based on our observations, the anti-psychiatric approach to therapy is unlikely to be suitable for patients with an epileptoid personality profile and a full-fledged epileptoid disorder due to their inclination towards a more orthodox view of the therapist's work. The epileptoid individual often seeks to see the therapist as a bastion of basic social values that they themselves occasionally ignore. Within society, the epileptoid personality is in a constant state of transition, first engaging in regretful actions and then seeking redemption through specific social institutions, often of a religious nature. Due to this dynamic, the therapist's indulgence in the various negative behavioral manifestations of the epileptoid personality is rarely perceived by the patient in a constructive manner. Therefore, we do not recommend the application of the anti-psychiatric approach in psychotherapy for patients with this personality profile due to its extremely low effectiveness.

Schizophrenic Profile

In fact, the anti-psychiatric approach was specifically developed in the 1950s and 1960s for patients with a schizophrenic personality profile. In this case, the most important aspect is the correctness and accuracy of the therapist's imitation strategy, which creates a mirror of the internal world of the schizophrenic patient. By correctness, we mean behavior with empathy that truly has a powerful healing effect on the patient. Excessive eccentricity in external behavioral forms can have a constructive effect but should not be the basis or the leading factor. The rules can be similar for patients with a schizophrenic accent. However, it is important to remember that deep adjustment through anti-psychiatric work is carried out to create new adaptive mechanisms in the patient's personality, which could potentially help them live more fully. This must be constantly taken into account and worked on, primarily through the prism of this belief.

Manic-Depressive Profile

Based on our observations, the anti-psychiatric approach is often not fully applicable to patients with MDP personality profile. The two key phases that patients go through—manic and depressive—often do not require reinforcement of the adequacy or inadequacy of their social manifestations. However, if we are discussing schizoaffective disorder, which can represent a specific combination of MDP and schizophrenic disorder, anti-psychiatric methods may find their place with proper and constructive application.

A Brief Message from the Author

Mastering complex psychotherapeutic theories and practices can be a challenging journey. By sharing your experience with this book, you can guide others who are on the same path. Your review could inspire someone to take the next step in deepening their knowledge and applying these insights to make meaningful changes in their life.

Thank you for your support and for taking the time to share your thoughts! Your feedback helps us refine our offerings and empowers others in their pursuit of mastering psychotherapy. If this book has been valuable to you, I'd be grateful if you could take a moment to leave a review. **Your positive rating would mean a lot!**

To share your feedback, simply scan the QR code or click the link below:

psychemaster.com/recommends/review-beyond-psychiatr y

Bibliography

1. Cooper, D. (1964). Reason and Violence: a decade of Sartre's philosophy. Tavistock.
2. Cooper, D. (1967). Psychiatry and Anti-Psychiatry (Ed.). Paladin.
3. Cooper, D. (1968). The Dialectics of Liberation (Ed.). Penguin.
4. Cooper, D. (1971). The Death of the Family. Penguin.
5. Cooper, D. (1974). Grammar of Living. Penguin.
6. Cooper, D. (1978). The Language of Madness. Penguin.
7. Laing, R. D. (1960). The Divided Self: An Existential Study in Sanity and Madness. Harmondsworth: Penguin.
8. Laing, R. D. (1961). The Self and Others. London: Tavistock Publications.
9. Laing, R. D., & Esterson, A. (1964). Sanity, Madness and the Family. Vol. 1. Families of Schizophrenics. London: Penguin Books.
10. Laing, R. D., & Cooper, D. G. (1964). Reason and Violence: A Decade of Sartre's Philosophy, 1950—1960. London: Tavistock Publications Ltd.
11. Laing, R. D. (1965). Mystification, Confusion and Conflict. In Boszormenyi-Nagy, I., and Framo, J. L. (eds.), Intensive Family Therapy. New York: Harper & Row.
12. Laing, R. D., Phillipson, H., & Lee, A. R. (1966). Inter-

personal Perception: A Theory and a Method of Research. London: Tavistock Publications, New York: Springer Pab. Co, 1966.

13. Laing, R. D. (1967). The Politics of Experience and the Bird of Paradise. Harmondsworth: Penguin.

14. Laing, R. D. (1970). Knots. London: Penguin.

15. Laing, R. D. (1971). The Politics of the Family and Other Essays. London: Tavistock Publications.

16. Laing, R. D. (1972). Knots. New York: Vintage Press.

17. Laing, R. D. (1976). The Facts of Life. London: Penguin.

18. Laing, R. D. (1977). Conversations with Adam and Natasha. New York: Pantheon.

19. Laing, R. D. (1978). Do You Love Me? An Entertainment in Conversation and Verse. New York: Penguin Books.

20. Laing, R. D. (1979). Sonnets. London: Michael Joseph.

21. Laing, R. D. (1982). The Voice of Experience: Experience, Science and Psychiatry. Harmondsworth: Penguin.

22. Laing, R. D. (1985). Wisdom, Madness and Folly: The Making of a Psychiatrist 1927—1957. London: Macmillan.

23. Laing, R. D. (1995). The Divided Self. Kyiv.

24. Laing, R. D. (1995). The Self and Others. Saint Petersburg: Belyy Krolik.

25. Laing, R. D. (2002). The "I" and Others. Moscow: Nezavisimaya firma "Klass."

26. Laing, R. D. (2002). I and Others. Knots. Moscow: Eksmo-Press.

27. Laing, R. D. (2005). Phenomenology of Experience. Lviv: Initsiativa.

28. Laing, R. D. (2012). Madness. Family Roots. BookMir.

29. Szasz, T. S. (1974). The Second Sin. Doubleday.

30. Szasz, T. S. (1975). The Age of Madness: A History of

Involuntary Mental Hospitalization Presented in Selected Texts. London: Routledge & Kegan Paul Ltd.

31. Szasz, T. S. (1988). Psychiatric Justice. Syracuse, New York: Syracuse University Press.

32. Szasz, T. S. (1988). The Ethics of Psychoanalysis: The Theory and Method of Autonomous Psychotherapy. Syracuse, New York: Syracuse University Press.

33. Szasz, T. S. (1988). Pain and Pleasure: A Study of Bodily Feelings. Syracuse, New York: Syracuse University Press.

34. Szasz, T. S. (1988). Schizophrenia: The Sacred Symbol of Psychiatry. Syracuse, New York: Syracuse University Press.

35. Szasz, T. S. (1988). The Theology of Medicine: The Political-Philosophical Foundations of Medical Ethics. Syracuse, New York: Syracuse University Press.

36. Szasz, T. S. (2001). Pharmacracy: Medicine and Politics in America. Westport CT: Praeger Publishers.

37. Szasz, T. S. (2002). Liberation By Oppression: A Comparative Study of Slavery and Psychiatry. New Brunswick, New Jersey: Transaction Publishers.

38. Szasz, T. S. (2004). Words to the Wise: A Medical-Philosophical Dictionary. New Brunswick, New Jersey: Transaction Publishers.

39. Szasz, T. S. (2008). Psychiatry: The Science of Lies. Syracuse, New York: Syracuse University Press.

40. Szasz, T. S. (2009). Antipsychiatry: Quackery Squared. Syracuse, New York: Syracuse University Press.

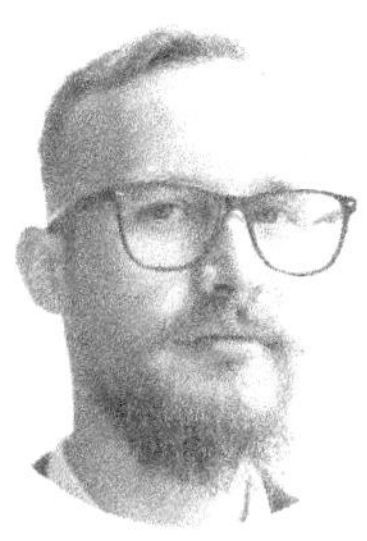

About the Author

Dr. **Artem Kudelia**, a psychologist with a PhD and a practicing therapist, has extensive expertise in integrative approaches. He possesses comprehensive knowledge of a wide range of psychotherapeutic methods, including humanistic and existential theories, as well as the practical application of cognitive-behavioral therapy (CBT) to effectively address issues such as anxiety, depression, obsessive thoughts, compulsions, social phobias, and complex emotions. His books are valuable resources for professionals and individuals interested in managing their mental health. In addition to managing symptoms, he helps his clients toward self-actualization in various aspects of their lives, including social, career, and personal aspects.

You can connect with me on:

- 🔗 https://facebook.com/psyche.masters
- 🔗 https://instagram.com/psyche.masters
- 🔗 https://threads.net/@psyche.masters
- 🔗 https://youtube.com/@psyche.masters
- 🔗 https://tiktok.com/@psyche.masters
- 🔗 https://pinterest.com/psychemasters

Subscribe to my newsletter:

- ✉ https://psychemaster.com/early-reader-signup

Also by Artem Kudelia PhD

The ***Psychology & Psychotherapy Theories & Practices*** series offers a detailed examination of the history, theoretical foundations, and practical applications of fundamental approaches in psychotherapy. It is an indispensable resource for psychologists, medical professionals, psychology students, and anyone interested in understanding these complex subjects.

Additionally, the ***Cognitive Behavioral Therapy Self-Help Guide: 15 Steps to Mental Health*** series provides actionable guidance for overcoming various psychological challenges, such as anxiety, depression, excessive anger, obsessive thoughts, compulsions, social phobias, health anxiety, and intricate emotional struggles. These topics were chosen because many individuals facing these challenges often lack awareness of the underlying dynamics. By gaining insight into these processes, individuals can make informed decisions about seeking help, reinforcing the idea that knowledge is a powerful tool for personal empowerment.

Together, these series offer invaluable resources for those interested in psychology, whether for academic study or personal development, by providing comprehensive insights and practical tools that contribute to improved mental well-being.

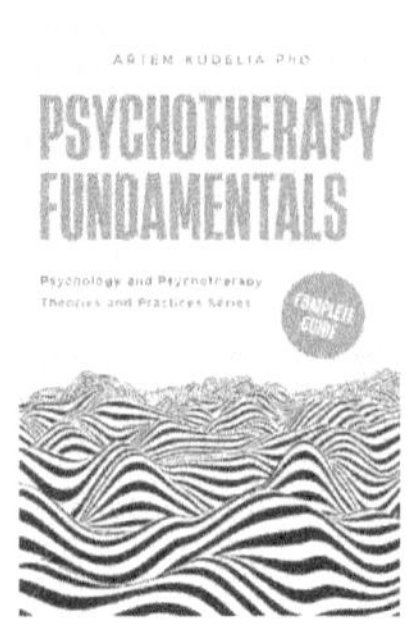

Psychotherapy Fundamentals Complete Guide

Are you struggling to understand complex psychotherapeutic theories?

Psychotherapy Fundamentals: Complete Guide simplifies the intricate world of psychotherapy, making it accessible and actionable for those interested in self-discovery, self-education, and readers with a wide range of interests.

💜 **Imagine confidently navigating psychotherapeutic real-world scenarios with ease.**

This book is your *comprehensive roadmap to achieving a deep and practical understanding of psychotherapy.* You'll learn to simplify complex theories and integrate them effectively into your life and practice.

Gain a comprehensive understanding of various therapeutic approaches, including *provocative* therapy, *humanistic* therapy, *somatic* therapy, *existential* therapy, *drama* therapy, *psychedelic* and *post-psychedelic* therapy, *anti-psychiatric* therapy, and *integrative* therapy. Each chapter delves into the key themes and methods of these psychotherapy modalities, broadening the horizons for those interested in self-discovery, self-education, and lifelong learning.

🔻

https://books2read.com/Psychotherapy-Fundamentals

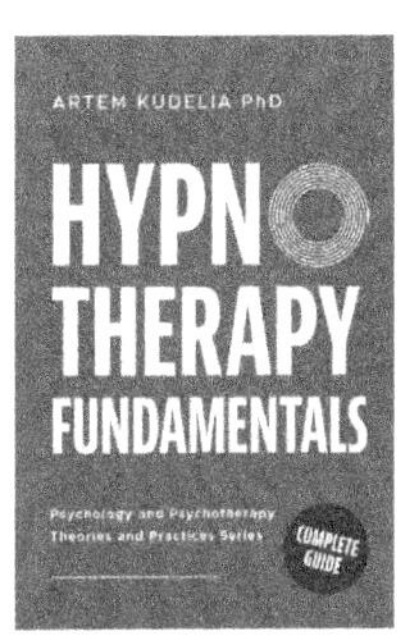

Hypnotherapy Fundamentals
Complete Guide

Are you ready to uncover the secrets of hypnotherapy?

This comprehensive guide immerses you in the **theory** *and history of hypnosis*, providing a solid foundation for understanding the principles underlying hypnotherapy.

Explore the various techniques and approaches used in *hypnotherapy* **training** through **practice exercises**, including the art of *suggestion* and deepening *hypnotic trance states*, the creation of therapeutic propositions, and the utilization of the power of the subconscious mind.

Learn how to effectively apply *hypnotherapy techniques* to address a wide range of issues, from managing stress and anxiety to overcoming phobias and habits.

Gain an understanding of the transformative potential of hypnosis and its applications for personal growth and well-being.

Unlock the secrets of harnessing the power of the mind and creating positive changes in yourself and others.

https://books2read.com/Hypnotherapy-Fundamentals

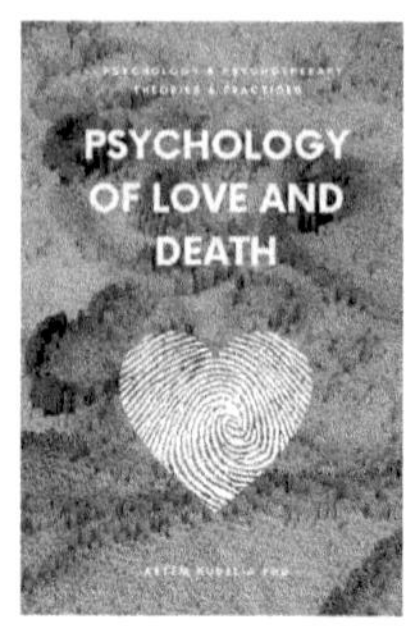

**Psychology of Love & Death
Therapeutic Path to Fundamental Balance
in Life and Relationships**

*How to Achieve Fundamental Balance in Life
and Relationships?*

Explore dualistic nature of human consciousness, along with the profound impact of seeking balance between fundamental continuums of *love and death, instinct and spirituality, masculinity and femininity* in shaping our experiences and relationships.

Explore the psychopathological profiles and manifestations of love and death, including profiles such as hysteria, paranoia, psychopathy, and others.

Uncover different types of love, from eros to agape, and study the *three-component Theory of Love.*

Familiarize yourself with *real-life psychotherapy cases* that illustrate the complexities of love, death, and therapy and gain *valuable insights* into the human experience and its challenges.

https://books2read.com/Psychology-of-Love-and-Death

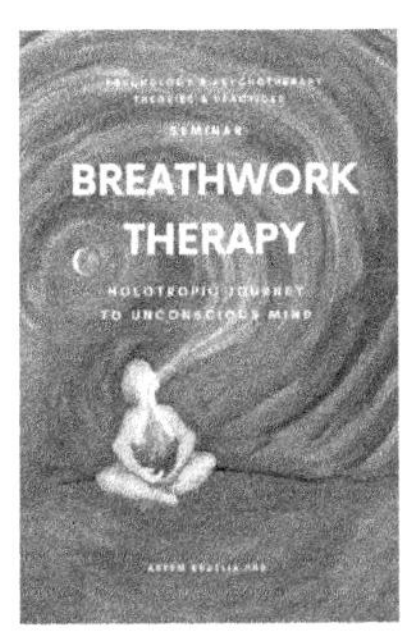

Breathwork Therapy Seminar Holotropic Journey to Unconscious Mind Secrets

Tap Into the Wisdom of Transpersonal Psychology!

This book is the transcript of a seminar that addresses the profound questions of *subconsciousness*, offering a unique perspective on personal growth and healing.

Gain profound insights into the workings of your mind and explore the mysteries of human consciousness.

Access practical exercises and *techniques* to facilitate personal growth, healing, and self-awareness through *breathwork*.

Written for seekers of self-awareness, psychology enthusiasts, and anyone curious about the depths of the human mind.

Explore the integration of spirituality and psychology, uncovering your inner potential.

https://books2read.com/Breathwork-Therapy

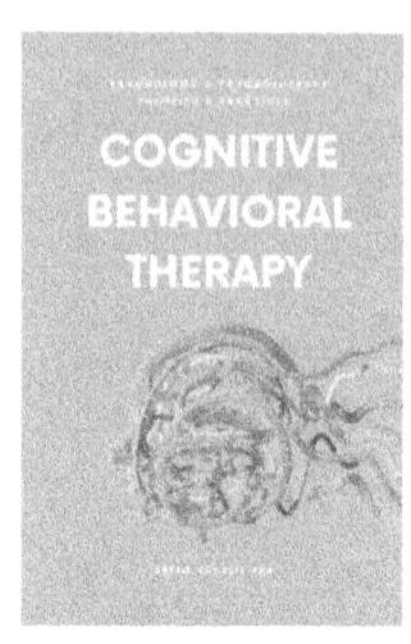

**Cognitive Behavioral Therapy
Managing Anxiety and Depression**

Explore the roots of anxiety and learn why it's a fundamental aspect of the human experience.

An in-depth exploration of *Panic Disorder*, addressing the irrational fears associated with it.

Examine the nuances of *Social Anxiety* and its impact on personal and professional spheres.

Dive into the world of *Obsessive-Compulsive Disorder*, unraveling its complexities.

Understand the genetic predispositions and learn effective strategies to manage obsessions and compulsions.

Explore *PTSD* from its roots to its biological manifestations. Delve into the trauma cycles, and discover therapeutic techniques for stabilization and overcoming trauma.

Grasp the degrees of *Depression*, from mild to severe, debunking common myths.

https://books2read.com/Cognitive-Behavioral-Therapy

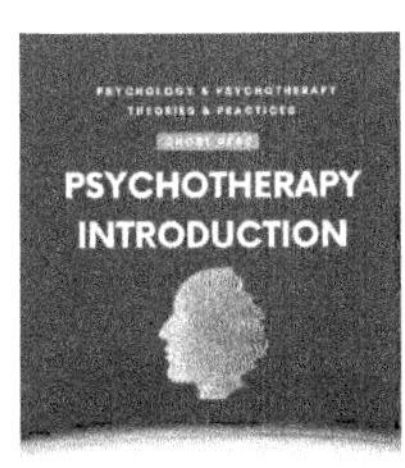

Psychotherapy
Introduction to Healing Vectors

Do you want to understand the variety of methods of psychotherapy and choose the one that is best for you?

In the vast world of psycho-technologies, there are numerous methods of psychotherapy that encompass a wide range of *personality theories* and concepts.

Drawing upon an integral framework, the book maps out the complex *landscape of psychotherapy*, encompassing vectors such as *psychoanalytic, hypnotic, provocative, humanistic, behavioral, existential, transpersonal, cognitive, somatic, psychodramatic* and *psychedelic* therapies, among many others.

This book will provide you with valuable knowledge that will allow you to choose the most suitable therapeutic path for specific circumstances and personality types.

https://books2read.com/Psychotherapy-Introduction

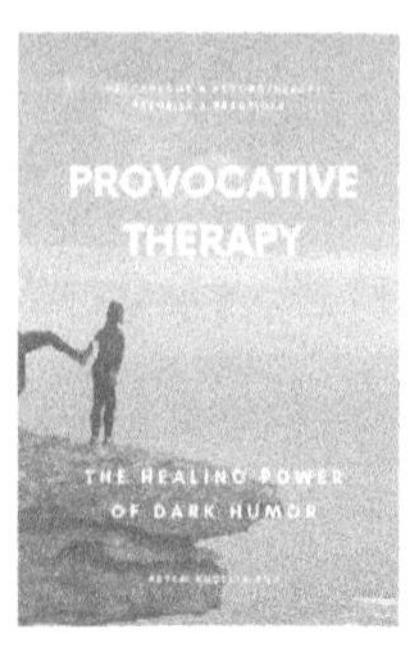

**Provocative Therapy
The Healing Power of Dark Humor**

Who said that psychotherapy can't be hilariously funny?

Explore innovative ideas about the power of humor in psychotherapy and coaching.

Uncover the archetypal foundation of Provocative Therapy inspired by the myths of the Trickster and the Holy Fool.

Delve into the transformational potential of *Group Provocative Psychotherapy* and the important rules that define successful group dynamics.

Explore the effectiveness of *Provocative Coaching* and its focus points.

Dive into the fascinating world of *Provocative Drama* and its role in therapeutic interventions.

Explore the *pathopsychological profiles*, including *hysteroid, paranoid, psychopathic, obsessive-compulsive, schizoid, epileptoid, schizophrenic,* and *manic-depressive* profiles.

https://books2read.com/Provocative-Therapy

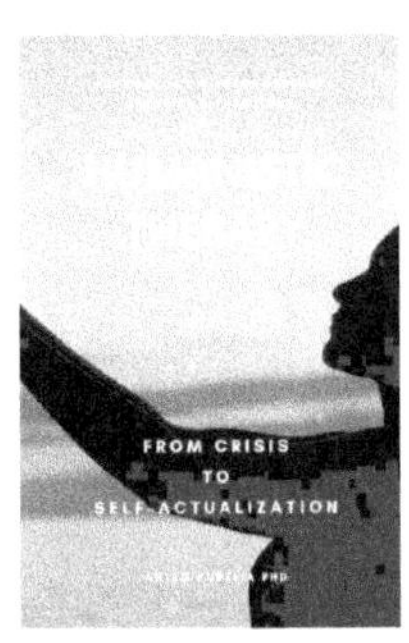

Humanistic Therapy
From Crisis to Self-Actualization

Do you want to explore a world where people are seen as unique holistic systems with infinite potential waiting to be discovered?

Immerse yourself in the theories and practices of humanistic therapy and explore the *transformative path from crisis to self-actualization.*

Unlike psychoanalysis, which focuses on internal complexes and personal traumas, humanistic therapy emphasizes the *study and development of positive personality qualities.*

Humanistic philosophy has also influenced fields such as *education*, promoting *empathy* and *support* as the foundation of learning.

This holistic approach recognizes the *interconnectedness of mind, body, and spirit* and seeks to stimulate personal *growth* and *well-being.*

Take the first step towards self-awareness, personal growth, and a more fulfilling existence.

https://books2read.com/Humanistic-Therapy

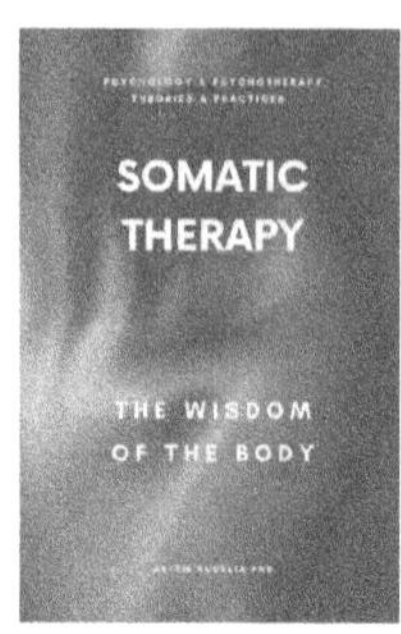

Somatic Therapy
The Wisdom of the Body

Would you like to establish a connection with your body and access the source of wisdom?

Unleash the transformative power of *somatic therapy* and embark on a journey of *self-discovery* and *healing.*

Explore the profound connection between the *mind and body.*

Discover the *seven levels of muscular armor* and their connection to specific emotions such as sadness, anger, and fear.

By exploring different body segments, you will unlock *powerful techniques* for releasing pent-up emotions and promoting harmony throughout the organism. From *eye movements* and *jaw exercises* to *deep breathing* and *body movements*, this book offers *practical methods* for *accessing the wisdom of the body* and *restoring emotional balance.*

Acquire unique knowledge about *healing after birth trauma and psychosomatic medicine.*

https://books2read.com/Somatic-Therapy

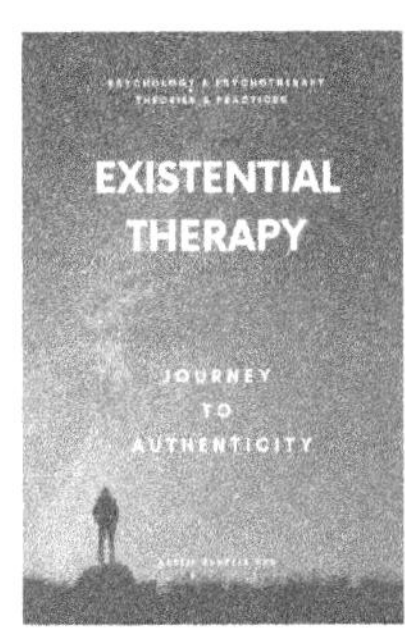

**Existential Therapy
Journey to Authenticity**

Do you want to know who you really are? What is your personal meaning of existence?

Embark on a *transformative journey* to uncover your *true essence* and embrace the *principles* of existential therapy.

Explore the rich philosophical roots of *existential psychotherapy* and find your path to *personal authenticity.*

Explore key themes such as *freedom, responsibility, meaning,* and *choice*, and learn to courageously and authentically navigate the complexities of existence.

This book provides *practical ideas and techniques* for *applying the principles of existential therapy* to your own life.

Gain a deep *understanding* of your *values, beliefs,* and *desires,* and learn to *embrace uncertainty* and *transform* life's *challenges* into *opportunities* for *growth* and *self-discovery.*

https://books2read.com/Existential-Therapy

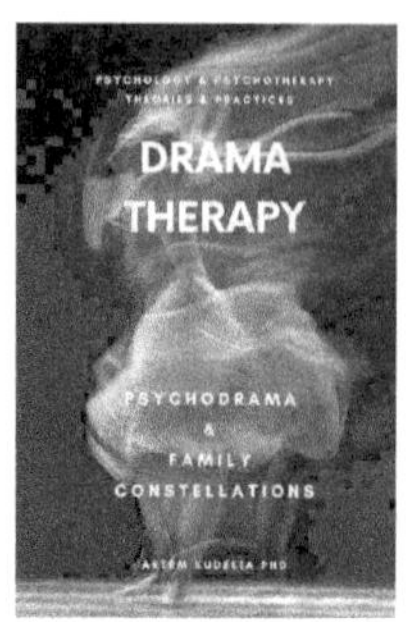

Drama Therapy
Potential of Psychodrama and Family Constellations

Explore the unique world of drama therapeutic approach!

Therapeutic model of intervention that encompasses *12 powerful speech patterns* capable of significantly *influencing conscious and unconscious processes.*

Through *psychodramatic techniques* and *family constellations*, you will *gain practical knowledge* to enhance your therapeutic practice.

Addressing a wide spectrum of *psychopathological profiles*, including *hysteria, paranoia,* and *obsessive-compulsive disorders*, this book equips you with effective dramatherapeutic activities and psychodynamic exercises.

It serves as a *comprehensive guide* to *crisis intervention, counseling theory*, and *strategies for addiction rehabilitation.*

Gain an understanding of the right hemisphere and the *neuroscience* underlying drama therapy, and learn to *navigate complex emotional situations* with *understanding* and *acceptance.*

https://books2read.com/Drama-Therapy-Constellations

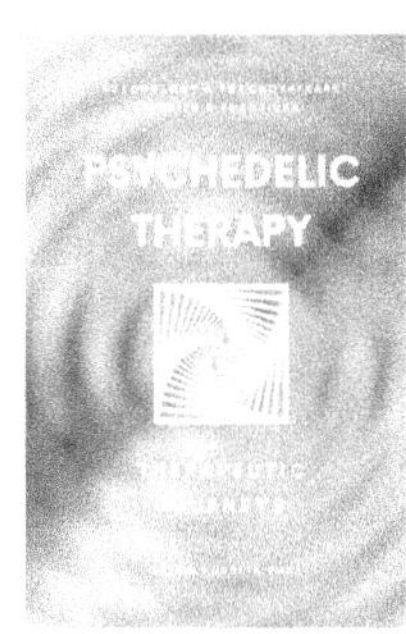

**Psychedelic Therapy
The Healing Power Therapeutic Journeys**

Embark on a transformative journey into the world of psychedelic therapy!

Explore the fascinating *history* of *psychedelic substances* and potential benefits of working with consciousness-altering substances in clinical practice.

Learn comprehensive information on various *psychedelic therapies*, including *ketamine therapy, psilocybin*-assisted psychotherapy, *MDMA*-assisted psychotherapy, and *ibogaine* psychotherapy.

Gain knowledge about *mental health* in the *perinatal period*, the *role of hypnosis*, and the transformative power of *holotropic breathwork*.

Understand the profound impact of *psychedelic medicine* and the potential of *psilocybin microdosing*.

Explore the therapeutic applications of *ketamine* in the *treatment of depression* and *psychosynthesis in coaching*.

https://books2read.com/Psychedelic-Therapy-Journey

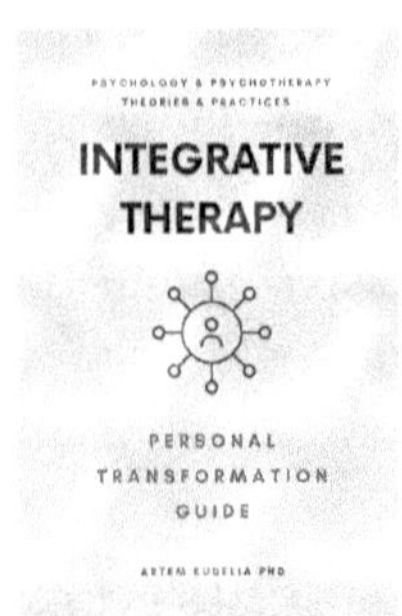

**Integrative Therapy
Personal Transformation Guide**

Discover the Power of Integrative Therapy and Embark on a Journey of Personal Transformation!

This book challenges traditional divisions in *therapeutic approaches* and explores the potential of *combining multiple vectors* to create a *comprehensive and integrated therapeutic system.*

Immerse yourself in the world of *neuro-linguistic programming* (NLP), *cognitive styles, neurological levels,* and *integral philosophy,* among other concepts.

Explore practical methodologies such as *shifting negative thinking, creating rapport,* and using linguistic patterns to facilitate positive change.

Unlock the transformative *power of anchors, changing personal history* and *submodalities.*

Gain an understanding of maps of the world and the *metamodel* for *effective communication.*

https://books2read.com/Integrative-Therapy

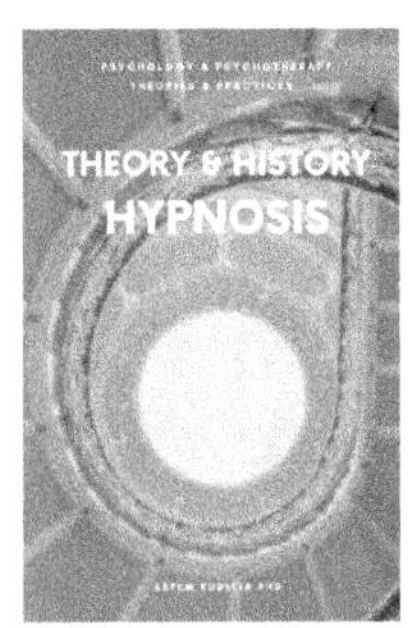

Theory & History of Hypnosis
Exploring Altered State of Mind in Trance

Immerse yourself in the fascinating world of hypnosis and explore the history and theory of altered states of consciousness!

This book sheds light on *historical trance practices* and the *role of shamanism*, tracing its influence on *modern psychospiritual orientations.*

Discover the benefits of this book by exploring the *history of trance practices and hypnotherapy.*

Explore the *evolution* of *shamanism*, its connection to *religion*, and its pre-religious *philosophy*, which offered deep insights into the structure of the universe and the mysteries of the spiritual world.

Discover various *hypnotic phenomena* and *states of consciousness* that can be induced in a trance state.

Explore their potential applications in *psychotherapeutic practice*, from *pain management* to the *treatment of depression.*

Learn techniques such as *self-hypnosis, deep trance induction*, and *guided healing visualizations.*

https://books2read.com/Theory-and-History-of-Hypnosis

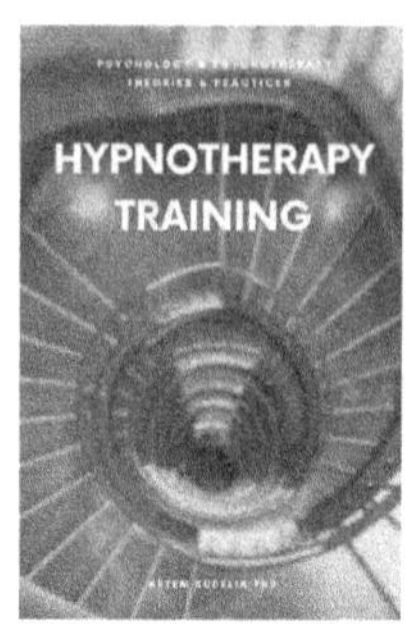

Hypnotherapy Training
A Guide for Practicing Hypnotherapists

Uncover the secrets of hypnotherapy and improve your practical hypnosis skills!

This book explores *techniques* and *practical skills* for hypnotherapists.

Dive into the depths of the *subconscious* and discover the *transformative potential* of hypnotherapy.

Discover the benefits of this book, which delves into key topics and approaches in *hypnotherapy training.*

Explore developed techniques, including rapport-building practices and the use of matching postures, movements, and breathing with the client.

Engage in exercises that enable the attainment of different trance levels and explore the motives of trance and their application in psychotherapy.

Gain an understanding of different styles and orientations of hypnotic work, from hypnoanalytic and suggestive to behavioral and transpersonal.

https://books2read.com/Hypnotherapy-Training

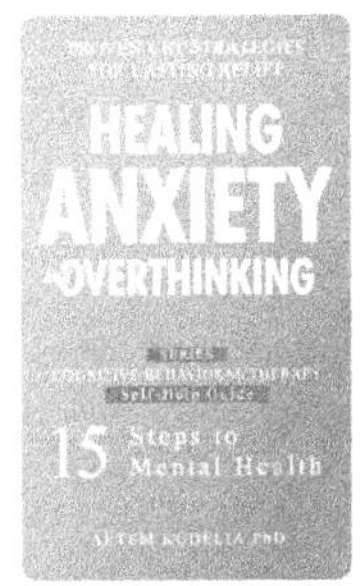

**Healing Anxiety and Overthinking
Proven CBT Strategies for Lasting Relief**

Are you exhausted from the relentless cycle of anxiety and overthinking?

Discover the 15-step program that will transform your mental health and bring peace of mind.

Millions of adults struggle with anxiety and overthinking, feeling trapped in a cycle of worry and stress. But it doesn't have to be this way. *"Healing Anxiety and Overthinking: Proven CBT Strategies for Lasting Relief"* offers a comprehensive guide to breaking free from the grip of anxiety using practical, proven **Cognitive Behavioral Therapy (CBT)** strategies.

💜 *Imagine waking up every day with a clear mind, free from the constant barrage of anxious thoughts*

This book is your roadmap to achieving that transformation in just 15 steps. You'll learn to understand the nature of your anxiety, identify its triggers, and apply effective techniques to manage and overcome it.

Take Control of Your Mental Health

Don't let anxiety and overthinking rule your life. With *"Healing Anxiety and Overthinking,"* you'll gain the tools and confidence to achieve peace of mind and live the life you deserve.

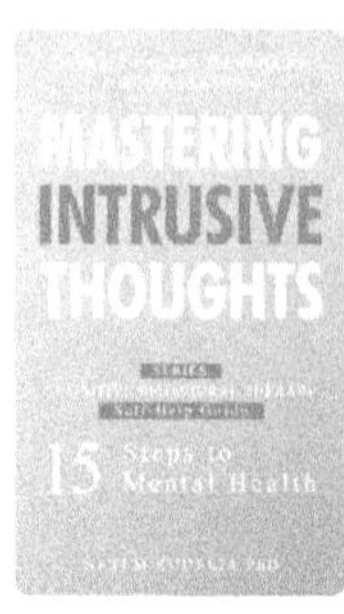

**Mastering Intrusive Thoughts
Practical CBT Techniques for Managing OCD**

*Is **OCD** ruling your life with intrusive thoughts and compulsions?*

Take back control with scientifically-proven CBT techniques designed to help you regain peace of mind.

Millions of adults struggle with obsessive-compulsive disorder (OCD), caught in a relentless cycle of intrusive thoughts and compulsive behaviors. "Mastering Intrusive Thoughts" is your step-by-step guide to breaking free from the grip of OCD using practical, evidence-based Cognitive Behavioral Therapy (CBT) techniques.

💜 *Picture yourself waking up with a calm, focused mind, no longer burdened by the constant anxiety of unwanted thoughts.*

In this book, Dr. Artem Kudelia offers a clear and actionable path to mastering your thoughts in 15 manageable steps. Whether you're new to CBT or have tried other methods without success, this guide provides the tools you need to finally achieve relief.

✔ **Take the First Step Towards Mental Freedom**

You'll gain the knowledge and confidence to conquer your **OCD** and reclaim your peace of mind.

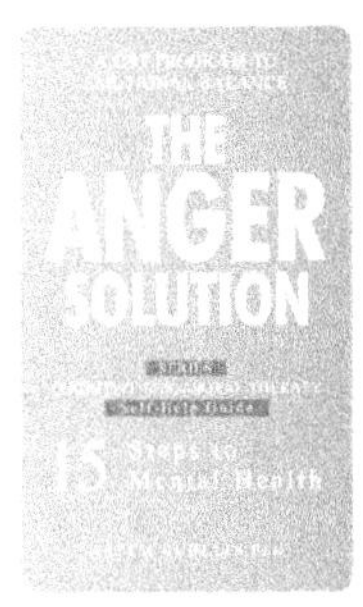

The Anger Solution
A CBT Program for Emotional Balance

Are you tired of living with persistent anger and overwhelming stress?

Discover a practical, 15-step program designed to bring lasting peace and transform your emotional health.

Millions of adults struggle with anger and stress, feeling trapped in a cycle of frustration and tension. But it doesn't have to be this way. "The Anger Solution" offers a comprehensive guide to breaking free from the grip of anger using practical, proven Cognitive Behavioral Therapy (CBT) strategies.

💜 *Imagine waking up every day with a calm mind, free from the constant barrage of anger and stress.*

This book is your roadmap to achieving that transformation. With clear, actionable steps, you'll learn to understand the nature of your anger, identify its triggers, and apply effective techniques to manage and overcome it.

✔ **Take Control of Your Emotional Health**

With "The Anger Solution," you'll gain the tools and confidence to achieve emotional balance and live the life you deserve.

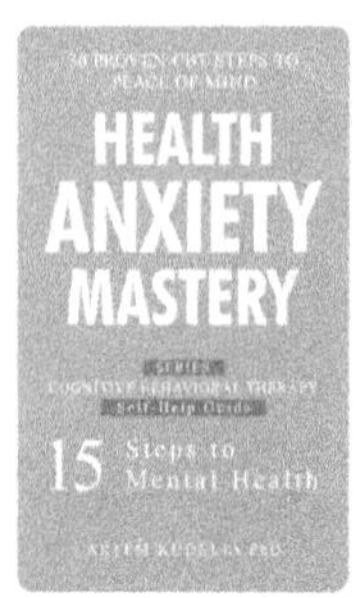

Health Anxiety Mastery
30 Proven CBT Steps to Peace of Mind

Is health anxiety controlling your life with constant worry and fear?

Regain peace of mind with proven CBT techniques designed to help you overcome health-related anxiety and reclaim control.

Millions of people struggle with health anxiety, trapped in a cycle of physical symptoms, endless reassurance-seeking, and intrusive thoughts about their well-being. *"Health Anxiety Mastery"* offers a clear, step-by-step approach to breaking free from these patterns using practical, evidence-based Cognitive Behavioral Therapy (CBT) techniques.

♥ **Imagine waking up each day calm and confident, no longer overwhelmed by fear and obsessive thoughts about your health.**

In this book, you'll find 30 actionable steps to help you reduce anxiety, challenge limiting beliefs, and develop healthier thought patterns. Whether you're just beginning your journey or have tried other approaches without success, these practical tools will guide you toward lasting relief.

✔ **Start Your Journey to Balanced Mental Health**

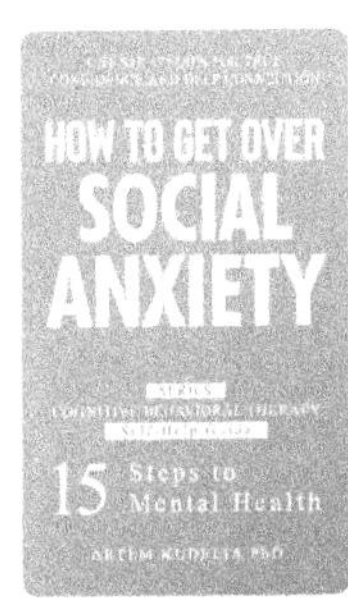

**How to Get Over Social Anxiety
CBT Strategies for True Confidence and
Deep Connection**

*What if 15 proven steps could free you from
social anxiety and help you connect?*

Uncover a 15-step CBT program to overcome
fear, stop avoidance, and build true self-
confidence. Millions struggle with social
anxiety, but you don't have to face it alone. This guide provides
a clear, evidence-based path to transforming your social life
and connecting authentically.

♥ **Imagine engaging in conversations fearlessly and forming
genuine relationships free from judgment or rejection.**

With insights from proven cognitive-behavioral techniques
and relatable examples, this book offers the practical tools and
encouragement needed to face your fears and succeed socially.

✔ **Begin Your Journey to Confidence**

Start transforming fear into connection and reclaim control of
your social life with **"*How to Get Over Social Anxiety*."**

Discover More by Artem Kudelia

Scan the QR code or click the link to access his author page and full collection. Each book provides detailed insights and practical guidance, exemplifying his contributions to psychology and psychotherapy.

books2read.com/Artem-Kudelia-PhD